VEGETABLES FOR GOOD HEALTH

A DIET RICH IN VEGETABLES AND FRUITS THAT LOWERS BLOOD PRESSURE

TABLE OF CONTENTS

Chapter One

What are vegetables and fruits

A vegetable is any edible portion of a plant. Vegetables are usually grouped according to the portion of the plant that is eaten such as leaves (lettuce), stem (celery), roots (carrot), tubers (potato), bulbs (onion) and flowers (broccoli). A fruit is the mature ovary of a plant.

A fruit is the matured ovary of a plant. So a tomato is botanically a fruit but is commonly considered a vegetable. According to this definition squash, pepper and eggplants are also fruits. Then there are seeds such as peas which are also considered vegetables.The edible product of a herbaceous plant-that is, a plant with a soft stem, as distinguished from the edible nuts and fruits produced by plants with woody stems such as shrubs and trees. Vegetables can be grouped according to the edible part of each plant: leaves (lettuce), stalks (celery), roots (carrot), tubers (potato), bulbs (onion), and flowers (broccoli). In addition, fruits such as the tomato and seeds such as the pea are commonly considered vegetables.

Commonly the term fruit is often restricted to succulent, edible fruits of woody plants, to melons, and to such small fruits as strawberries and blueberries. In nature, fruit is normally produced only after fertilization of ovules has taken place, but in many plants, largely cultivated varieties such as seedless citrus fruits, bananas, and cucumbers, fruit matures without fertilization, a process known as parthenocarpy. In either case, the maturation of the ovary results in the withering of stigmas and anthers and enlargement of the ovary or ovaries. Ovules within fertilized ovaries develop to produce seeds. In unfertilized varieties, seeds fail to develop, and the ovules remain their original size. The major service performed by fruit is the protection of developing seeds. In many plants, fruit also aids in seed distribution.

Vegetables can be eaten either raw or cooked and play an important role in human nutrition, being mostly low in fat and carbohydrates, but high in vitamins, minerals and dietary fiber. Many nutritionists encourage people to consume plenty of fruit and vegetables, five or more portions a day often being recommended.

Nowadays, most vegetables are grown all over the world as climate permits, and crops may be cultivated in protected environments in less suitable locations. China is the largest producer of vegetables, and global trade in agricultural products allows consumers to purchase vegetables grown in faraway countries. The scale of production varies from subsistence farmers supplying the needs of their family for food, to agribusinesses with vast acreages of single-product crops. Depending on the type of vegetable concerned, harvesting the crop is followed by grading, storing, processing, and marketing.

Chapter 2

Vegetables for a good health

There are some certain foods we should not consume that can be harmful to the body system and health, consuming a diet rich in vegetables, fruit, whole grains, nuts, seeds, and fish (and low in red meat, salt, and added sugars) may help lower blood pressure over time.

The foods and vegetables that helps to Lower blood pressure are:

- Leafy greens: which are high in potassium

Potassium helps your kidneys get rid of more sodium through your urine. This in turn lowers your blood pressure.

- Citrus fruits

Citrus fruits, including grapefruit, oranges, and lemons, may have powerful blood-pressure-lowering effects. They're loaded with vitamins, minerals, and plant compounds that may help keep your heart healthy by reducing heart disease risk factors like high blood pressure.

- Salmon and other fatty fish

Fatty fish are an excellent source of omega-3 fats, which have significant heart health benefits. These fats may help reduce blood pressure levels by reducing inflammation and decreasing levels of blood-vessel-constricting compounds called oxylipins.

- Pumpkin seeds may be small, but they pack a punch when it comes to nutrition.

They're a concentrated source of nutrients important for blood pressure control, including magnesium, potassium, and arginine, an amino acid needed for the production of nitric oxide, which is essential for blood vessel relaxation and blood pressure reduction.

Pumpkin seed oil has also been shown to be a powerful natural remedy for high blood pressure. A study in 23 women found that supplementing with 3 grams of pumpkin seed oil per day for 6 weeks led to significant reductions.

- Beans and lentils

Beans and lentils are rich in nutrients that help regulate blood pressure, such as fiber, magnesium, and potassium. Numerous studies have shown that eating beans and lentils may help lower high blood pressure levels.

- Berries

Berries have been associated with a variety of impressive health benefits, including their potential to reduce heart disease risk factors like high blood pressure. Berries are a rich source of antioxidants, including anthocyanins, which are pigments that give berries their vibrant color.Blueberries, raspberries, chokeberries, cloudberries, and strawberries are just some of the berries that have been associated with blood-pressure-lowering effects.

- Amaranth

Amaranth is a whole grain that's particularly high in magnesium. One cooked cup (246 grams) provides 38% of your daily magnesium needs.

Eating whole grains like amaranth may help lower your blood pressure levels. Studies show that diets rich in whole grains may decrease your risk of high blood pressure.

- Pistachios

Pistachios are highly nutritious, and their consumption has been linked to healthy blood pressure levels. They're high in a number of nutrients essential for heart health and blood pressure regulation, including potassium.

- Carrots

Crunchy, sweet, and nutritious, carrots are a staple veggie in many people's diets. Carrots are high in phenolic compounds, such as chlorogenic, p-coumaric, and caffeic acids, that help relax blood vessels and reduce inflammation, which may help lower blood pressure levels

Although carrots can be enjoyed cooked or raw, eating them raw may be more beneficial for reducing high blood pressure.

- Tomatoes and tomato products

Tomatoes and tomato products are rich in many nutrients, including potassium and the carotenoid pigment lycopene.

Lycopene has been significantly associated with beneficial effects on heart health, and eating foods high in this nutrient, such as tomato products, may help reduce heart disease risk factors like high blood pressure.

- Herbs and spices

Certain herbs and spices contain powerful compounds that may help reduce blood pressure by helping blood vessels relax.

Celery's seed, cilantro, saffron, lemongrass, black cumin, ginseng, cinnamon, cardamom, sweet basil, and ginger are just some of the herbs and spices that have been shown to have blood-pressure-lowering potential, according to results from animal and human research.

- Spinach

Like beets, spinach is high in nitrates. It's also loaded with antioxidants, potassium, calcium, and magnesium, making it an excellent choice for people with high blood pressure.

The spinach soup also decreased artery stiffness, which may help reduce blood pressure and improve heart health.

Along with other lifestyle modifications, adopting a healthy diet can significantly lower blood pressure levels and help reduce your heart disease risk.

According to research, adding certain foods like leafy greens, berries, beans, lentils, seeds, fatty fish, citrus fruits, and carrots to your meals and snacks may help you reach and maintain optimal blood pressure levels.

If you have high blood pressure levels or are looking to maintain healthy blood pressure, adding a few of the foods listed in this article to your diet may help.

Chapter three

Important of fruits and vegetables

Fruit and vegetables should be an important part of your daily diet. They are naturally good and contain vitamins and minerals that can help to keep you healthy. They can also help protect against some diseases.

Most Australians will benefit from eating more fruit and vegetables as part of a well-balanced, regular diet and a healthy, active lifestyle. There are many varieties of fruit and vegetables available and many ways to prepare, cook and serve them.

You should eat at least five serves of vegetables and two serves of fruit each day. Choose different colours and varieties.

A serve of vegetables is about one cup of raw salad vegetables or 1/2 cup of cooked.

A serve of fruit is about one medium piece, 2 small pieces of 1 cup canned (no added sugar).

Chapter four

Types of vegetables

Vegetables are available in many varieties and can be classified into biological groups or 'families', including:

Leafy green – lettuce, spinach and silverbeet
Cruciferous – cabbage, cauliflower, Brussels sprouts and broccoli
Marrow – pumpkin, cucumber and zucchini
Root – potato, sweet potato and yam
Edible plant stem – celery and asparagus
Allium – onion, garlic and shallot.
Legumes

- Legumes or pulses contain nutrients that are especially valuable. Legumes need to be cooked before they are eaten – this improves their nutritional quality, aids digestion and eliminates any harmful toxins. Legumes come in many forms including:

Soy products – tofu (bean curd) and soybeans
Legume flours – chickpea flour (besan), lentil flour and soy flour
Dried beans and peas – haricot beans, red kidney beans, chickpeas and lentils
Fresh beans and peas – green peas, green beans, butter beans, broad beans and snow peas.

Chapter five

Preparations of some vegetables and fruits

Vegetables are often cooked, although some kinds are eaten raw. Cooking and processing can damage some nutrients and phytochemicals in plant foods.

Suggestions to get the best out of your fruit and vegetables include:
.Eat raw vegetables and fruits if possible.
Try fruit or vegetables pureed into smoothies.
Use a sharp knife to cut fresh fruits to avoid bruising.
Cut off only the inedible parts of vegetables – sometimes the best nutrients are found in the skin, just below the skin or in the leaves.
Use stir-fry, grill, microwave, bake or steam methods with non-stick cookware and mono-unsaturated oils.
Do not overcook, to reduce nutrient loss.
Serve meals with vegetable pestos, salsas, chutneys and vinegars in place of sour cream, butter and creamy sauces.
Some nutrients such as carotenoids may actually be increased if food is cooked. For example, tomato has more carotenoids, especially lycopene, when it is cooked – a good reason to prepare fruits and vegetables in a variety of ways.

Once you've prepared and cooked your vegetables and fruit, spend some time on presentation. People are more likely to enjoy a meal if it's full of variety and visually appealing, as well as tasty. Sit at the table to eat and enjoy your food without distractions like television.

Chapter six

Vegetables for family health

vegetable serving suggestions for your family's health
Vegetables and fruit are a handy snack food and are easily carried to work or school. Include them in everyone's meals and snacks for a healthy, well-balanced diet. Some suggestions include:

.Keep snack-size fruit and vegetable portions easily accessible in your fridge.
.Keep fresh fruit on the bench or table.
.Add fruit and vegetables to your favourite family recipes or as additions to your usual menus.
Use the colour and texture of a variety of fruit and vegetables to add interest to your meals.
Think up new ways to serve fruits and vegetables.
Some simple ways to serve fruits and vegetables include:
fruit and vegetable salads
vegetable or meat-and-vegetable stir-fries
raw fruit and vegetables
vegetable soups
snack pack, stewed or canned fruits or dried fruits.
Limit fruit juice, as it does not contain the same amount of nutrients as fresh fruit. It also contains a lot of sugars. These sugars are not necessarily good for your health, even though they are 'natural'. Instead, have a drink of water and a serve of fruit.

Chapter Seven

Tips to lower blood pressure

Here are some great tips helps lower your overall blood pressure, including diastolic blood pressure.

- Focus on heart-healthy foods

Foods that are an integral part of a heart-healthy diet include:
VEGETABLES such as spinach, broccoli, and carrots
FRUITS such as apples, oranges, and bananas
Fish, particularly those rich in omega-3 fatty acids
lean cuts of beef or pork
skinless chicken or turkey
eggs
fat-free or low-fat dairy products, such as cheese and yogurt
whole grains, such as brown rice and whole-grain bread
nuts and beans

- Limit saturated and trans fats

Try not to eat foods that are high in saturated or trans fats. Examples include fast food, hot dogs, and frozen food.

Instead, try to focus on consuming healthy monounsaturated and polyunsaturated fats that can be found in things like avocados, olive or canola oil, and nuts.

- Reduce sodium in your diet

Sodium can increase blood pressure, so limit your intake to 1,500 milligrams or less per day.

- Eat more potassium

Potassium can actually counteract the effect that sodium has on your blood pressure.Trusted Source Try to boost consumption of foods rich in potassium, such as bananas, spinach, and tomatoes.

- Lay off the caffeine

Caffeine is a stimulant that can raise blood pressure. If you have hypertension, try to limit your intake, particularly before activities that can raise blood pressure, such as exercise.

- Cut back on alcohol

Drinking excess alcohol can raise your blood pressure. Consume it in moderation. That means two drinks per day for men and one drink per day for women.

- Ditch sugar

Foods with added sugars can add calories to your diet that you don't need. Avoid foods and drinks that contain added sugars or sweeteners, such as soft drinks, cakes, and candies.

- Reduce stress

Stress is another thing that can raise your blood pressure. Try to avoid things that trigger stress. Practicing activities such as meditation or deep breathing may also help lower stress.

- Stop smoking

The nicotine in cigarettes is a stimulant that can increase your blood pressure. It can also lead to injury of the walls of your blood vessels. Not only is quitting smoking beneficial for your overall health, but it can also help lower your blood pressure.

- Try supplements

Although more research may be needed, some studies show that supplements such as garlic can help lower blood pressure.

Chapter Eight
Some foods to avoid

Here are some certain foods we should always avoid. Foods high in salt, sugar, and saturated or trans fats can increase blood pressure and damage your heart health. By limiting these foods and replacing them with healthy options, you can keep your blood pressure at a healthy level.Highly processed foods, saturated fats, salt, fried food, and excessive alcohol intake should be avoided. These can elevate blood pressure.
Exceeding your recommended daily calorie intake is also bad for your blood pressure. Too many calories causes weight gain. "Excess weight elevates blood pressure.
SOME FOODS THAT MAY RISE BLOOD PRESSURE:
.Processed meats such as bacon and hot dogs
.Canned foods with preservatives
.High-sodium foods such as pickles and potato chips
.Fried foods such as french fries and chicken strips
.Fatty meats
.Vegetable oil and margarine, which are high in trans fat
.Table salt
.Grapefruit*
Consuming nitrate-rich vegetables can help lower blood pressure for up to 24 hours. This lowering may not bring blood pressure into the normal range. It is important to check your blood pressures at home, and at the grocery store or pharmacy with the goal of less than 135/85. Nitrate-rich vegetables should not be confused with nitrate-rich foods laden with preservatives.
When most people hear nitrate, the first thing they think of is processed meat because artificial nitrate is added to bacon, hot dogs, and salami for preservation. "When taken from animal sources, nitrate is converted into carcinogenic nitrosamine in your body, which is extremely harmful to your health," Dr. Lam says. Nitrates from vegetables, fruits, and grains on the other hand are converted to nitric oxide in your body. Nitric oxide helps relax blood vessels and improves blood flow.
While there is no single food that you can eat to lower your blood pressure, a healthy eating plan that incorporates all of the necessary components can help. "It includes adequate cereal fiber from grains, and other fibers from fruits, vegetables and legumes.
Whole grains provide minerals such as magnesium, which works with the calcium in low-fat dairy to improve your health. Fruit and vegetables provide potassium. Potassium reduces the effect of sodium and decreases the tension in your blood vessels. These are all important to maintain good health and maximize blood pressure control.

Chapter Nine

Foods that triggers blood pressure and some health issues

- Table Salt

If you are trying to follow a low-sodium diet, this seems like an obvious one, but it needs to be said. A lot of people reach for the salt shaker by habit when preparing meals and snacks, but it should be very limited or avoided altogether when dealing with high blood pressure. Find new spices and herbs to use to flavor dishes.

- Certain Condiments and Sauces

When replacing table salt, do not fall into the trap of substituting certain condiments instead. Things like ketchup, soy sauce, salad dressing, barbecue sauce, and steak sauce all have a lot of sodium in them. Other places salt can be hidden is in pasta sauce and gravy. Familiarize yourself with different herbs and spices to add flavor to foods instead.

- Foods with Saturated and Trans Fat

There are healthy fats you can have in your diet even with high blood pressure, but saturated and trans fats are not among them. Things fried in a lot of oils or meats that have a lot of fat are bad for both blood pressure and cholesterol.

Reduce or eliminate red meat consumption. If you do eat red meat, make sure you read labels and choose the leanest cuts possible.

If you consume a lot of dairy, switch to low-fat versions. And be careful of cheeses with high salt content.

- Fried Food

Fried foods contain a lot of saturated fat and salt, both of which you should avoid when you have high blood pressure. Grilling, baking, and sautéing are all good alternatives to frying. Air-fryers have become popular and are a good option as long as you pay attention to the salt content of what you're cooking in the first place. Any kind of breading or seasoning mixes should be low sodium.

- Fast Food

If you're following any kind of nutritional guidelines, fast food is a bad idea all-around. A lot of the food served at fast-food restaurants is processed and frozen, then cooked by frying or cooking in high-fat oils. Additionally, they are often heavily salted. Because these are foods that increase blood pressure, they should be avoided.

- Canned, Frozen, and Processed Foods

These foods can be convenient, however, many of them contain large amounts of added salt to preserve flavor through the canning, packaging, or freezing process.

- Salted Snacks

Many crackers, chips, and even sweets like cookies, are not good options. Other things to look out for include jerky and nuts. Those might seem like healthier snacks because they are sources of protein and healthy fats (in certain nuts), but for those with high blood pressure, they can be bad news. Look for varieties with no or very little salt added. Another good option if you are craving a crunchy snack, is popping your own plain popcorn and adding (salt-free) spices to it yourself.

You should also avoid pickled foods, which are often full of salt as a result of the pickling process. Most pickling processes use a lot of salt in the brine mixture to kill bacteria, and the sodium sticks around after the pickling is done.

- Caffeine

Coffee, tea, energy drinks, and soda all contain caffeine, which is known to increase blood pressure. People with hypertension should limit their caffeine intake. If you are a coffee lover, try switching to half-caff coffee, or decaf if you can't give it up completely. There are also caffeine-free teas available and certain varieties of tea have very low amounts of caffeine naturally.

- Alcohol

Small amounts of alcohol have been found to lower blood pressure, but drinking too much can increase it.

Eating certain types of food can help you raise your blood pressure. Monitor your symptoms and regularly measure your blood pressure to see what works. Try to consume:

More fluids. Dehydration decreases blood volume, causing blood pressure to drop. Staying hydrated is especially important when exercising.

Foods high in vitamin B-12. Too little vitamin B-12 can lead to a certain type of anemia, which can cause low blood pressure and fatigue. Foods high in B-12 include eggs, fortified cereals, animal meats, and nutritional yeast.

Foods high in folate. Too little folate can also contribute to anemia. Examples of folate-rich foods include asparagus, beans, lentils, citrus fruits, leafy greens, eggs, and liver.

Salty foods can increase blood pressure. Try eating canned soup, smoked fish, cottage cheese, pickled items, and olives.

Caffeine. Coffee and caffeinated tea may temporarily spike blood pressure by stimulating the cardiovascular system and boosting your heart rate.

Chapter Ten

Daily allowances of fruit and vegetables

There are different fruits and vegetables that contains different nutrients. The Australian dietary guidelines recommend that adults eat at least five kinds of vegetable and two kinds of fruit every day. A national nutrition survey conducted by the Australian Government showed that Australians of all ages do not eat enough vegetables and fruit.

Children have a smaller stomach capacity and higher energy needs than adults. They cannot eat the same serving sizes as adults. However, you should encourage your children to eat a variety of fruits and vegetables. By eating well, your children will have the energy they need to play, concentrate better, learn, sleep better and build stronger teeth and bones. Building good habits in their early years can also provide the protection of a healthy diet throughout their lives.

Chapter Eleven
Legumes benefits in health

Legumes are fiber-rich plant-based foods that include beans, lentils, and peas.
Beans are a good source of fermentable fibers. This fiber moves into the large intestine and helps to feed the diverse colony of healthy bacteria in the gut.
Researchers have found connections Trusted Source between a healthy gut microbiome and lower rates of obesity and type 2 diabetes.

The following are some of the best legumes for fiber:

- Navy beans

Navy beans are one of the richest sources of fiber. They are also high in protein. Add navy beans to salads, curries, or stews for an extra fiber and protein boost.

Fiber content: Navy beans contain 10.5 g per 100 gTrusted Source (31.3 percent of AI).

- Pinto Beans

Pinto beans are a popular U.S. staple. People can eat pinto beans whole, mashed or as refried beans. Along with their high-fiber content, pinto beans are a great source of calcium and iron.
Fiber content: Pinto beans contain 9 g of fiber per 100 gTrusted Source (26.8 percent of AI).

- Black beans

Black beans contain good amounts of iron and magnesium. They are also a great source of plant-based protein.

If people who follow a vegan diet combine black beans with rice, they will be getting all nine essential amino acids.
Fiber content: Black beans contain 8.7 g of fiber per 100 gTrusted Source (25.9 percent of AI).

- Split peas

Split peas are a great source of iron and magnesium. They go well in casseroles, curries, and dahl.
Fiber content: Split peas contain 8.3 g of fiber per 100 gTrusted Source (24.7 percent of AI).

- Lentils

There are many types of lentils, including red lentils and French lentils. They make a great addition to couscous, quinoa dishes, or dahl.
Fiber content: Lentils contain 7.9 g of fiber per 100 gTrusted Source (23.5 percent of AI).

- Mung beans

Mung beans are a versatile source of potassium, magnesium, and vitamin B-6.

When dried and ground, people can use mung bean flour to make pancakes.
Fiber content: Mung beans contain 7.6 g of fiber per 100 gTrusted Source (22.6 percent of AI).

- Adzuki beans

Adzuki beans are used in Japanese cuisine to make red bean paste, which is a traditional sweet. People can also boil these fragrant, nutty beans and eat them plain.
Fiber content: Adzuki beans contain 7.3 g of fiber per 100 gTrusted Source (21.7 percent of AI).

- Lima Beans

Not only are lima beans a great source of fiber, but they are also high in plant protein.
Fiber content: Lima beans contain 7 g of fiber per 100 gTrusted Source (20.8 percent of AI).

- Chickpeas

Chickpeas, or garbanzo beans, are a popular source of plant-based protein and fiber. They are also full of iron, vitamin B-6, and magnesium.

Use this legume as a base for hummus and falafel.

Fiber content:
Legumes
Vegetables
Fruit
Nuts and seeds
Whole grains
Tips to increase fiber in the diet
Summary
When a person includes high-fiber foods in their diet, it has many benefits, such as keeping the gut healthy, boosting heart health, and promoting weight loss.

According to the most up-to-date Dietary Guidelines for AmericansTrusted Source, the adequate intake of fiber for adult men is 33.6 (g) per day, and 28 g for adult women.
But most people in America do not meet this goal. The average fiber intake in the United States is 17 g, and only 5 percent of people meet the adequate daily intake.
People need to get both soluble and insoluble fiber from their diet. Eating a varied high-fiber diet means getting plenty of fruits, vegetables, legumes, and whole grains.

In this article, we provide a list of 38 healthful, high-fiber foods explaining how much fiber each one has to help people boost their daily fiber intake.

High-fiber legumes
Navy beans contain 10.5 g of fiber per 100 g and are also high in protein.
Legumes are fiber-rich plant-based foods that include beans, lentils, and peas.

Beans are a good source of fermentable fibers. This fiber moves into the large intestine and helps to feed the diverse colony of healthy bacteria in the gut.

Researchers have found connections Trusted Source between a healthy gut microbiome and lower rates of obesity and type 2 diabetes.

The following are some of the best legumes for fiber:

- Navy beans

Navy beans are one of the richest sources of fiber. They are also high in protein. Add navy beans to salads, curries, or stews for an extra fiber and protein boost.

Fiber content: Navy beans contain 10.5 g per 100 gTrusted Source (31.3 percent of AI).

- Pinto Beans

Pinto beans are a popular U.S. staple. People can eat pinto beans whole, mashed or as refried beans. Along with their high-fiber content, pinto beans are a great source of calcium and iron.

Fiber content: Pinto beans contain 9 g of fiber per 100 gTrusted Source (26.8 percent of AI).

- Black beans

Black beans contain good amounts of iron and magnesium. They are also a great source of plant-based protein.

If people who follow a vegan diet combine black beans with rice, they will be getting all nine essential amino acids.

Fiber content: Black beans contain 8.7 g of fiber per 100 gTrusted Source (25.9 percent of AI).

- Split peas

Split peas are a great source of iron and magnesium. They go well in casseroles, curries, and dahl.

Fiber content: Split peas contain 8.3 g of fiber per 100 gTrusted Source (24.7 percent of AI).

- Lentils

There are many types of lentils, including red lentils and French lentils. They make a great addition to couscous, quinoa dishes, or dahl.

Fiber content: Lentils contain 7.9 g of fiber per 100 g.

- Mung beans

Mung beans are a versatile source of potassium, magnesium, and vitamin B-6.

When dried and ground, people can use mung bean flour to make pancakes.

Fiber content: Mung beans contain 7.6 g of fiber per 100 g.

- Adzuki beans

Adzuki beans are used in Japanese cuisine to make red bean paste, which is a traditional sweet. People can also boil these fragrant, nutty beans and eat them plain.

Fiber content: Adzuki beans contain 7.3 g of fiber per 100 g.

- Lima Beans

Not only are lima beans a great source of fiber, but they are also high in plant protein.
Fiber content: Lima beans contain 7 g of fiber per 100 g.

- Chickpeas

Chickpeas, or garbanzo beans, are a popular source of plant-based protein and fiber. They are also full of iron, vitamin B-6, and magnesium.

Use this legume as a base for hummus and falafel.
Fiber content: Chickpeas contain 6.4 g of fiber per 100 g.

- Kidney Beans

Kidney beans are a rich source of iron. Kidney beans are a great addition to chili, casseroles, and salads.
Fiber content: Kidney beans contain 6.4 g of fiber per 100 g.

- Soybeans

Soybeans are used to make a variety of products, such as tofu, tempeh, and miso. People often use soybean products as dietary replacements for meat and dairy.

Fresh soybeans can also be eaten raw or added to salads as edamame.
Fiber content: Soybeans contain 6 g of fiber per 100 g.

- Baked beans

Baked beans are rich in fiber and protein. They are available from most grocery stores. Try to buy brands with reduced sugar and salt to get more health benefits.
Fiber content: Plain baked beans from a can contain 4.1 g of fiber per 100g.

- Green peas

Green peas are available canned or fresh. Green peas are a great source of fiber, protein, vitamin C, and vitamin A.
Fiber content: Green peas contain 4.1–5.5 g of fiber per 100 g.

High-fiber vegetables

Among the many health benefits of vegetables, they are a great source of dietary fiber. Vegetables with a high-fiber content include:

- Artichokes are packed with vitamins C and K, plus calcium, and folate.

Grill, bake, or steam whole artichokes and use in dishes or as a side.
People often prepare just the artichoke heart above the outside leaves.
Fiber content: One medium artichoke contains 6.9 g of fiber.

- Potato

As a staple vegetable, potatoes are a good source of B vitamins plus vitamin C and magnesium.
Fiber content: One large potato, baked in its skin, contains 6.3 g of fiberTrusted Source.

- Sweet potato

Sweet potatoes are one of the starchy vegetables. They are high in vitamin A.
Fiber content: One large sweet potato, baked in its skin, contains 5.9 g of fiberTrusted Source.

- Parsnips

Parsnips are a good source of vitamins C and K, as well as B vitamins, calcium, and zinc.
Fiber content: One boiled parsnip contains 5.8 g of fiber.

- Winter squash

Winter squash vegetables are a bountiful source of vitamins A and C.
Fiber content: One cup of winter squash contains 5.7 g of fiber.

- Broccoli

Broccoli is a cruciferous vegetable that is high in vitamins C and A. Cruciferous vegetables also have lots of antioxidant polyphenols.
Fiber content: One cup of cooked broccoli florets contains 5.1 g of fiber.

- Pumpkin

Pumpkin is a popular vegetable and source of vitamins A and K and calcium. People use it in sweet and savory dishes.
Fiber content: A standard portion of canned pumpkin contains 3.6 g of fiber.

High-fiber fruit
People can boost their daily fiber intake by including healthful fruits as a snack between meals. Some fruits contain more fiber than others.

- Avocado

Avocado is full of healthful monounsaturated fats that are beneficial to heart health. They are popular in salads and for making dips.
Fiber content: One peeled avocado contains 9.2 g of fiber.

- Pear

Pears are full of fiber, as well as vitamins C and A, folate and calcium. Keep a few pears in the fruit bowl, or serve them with dessert.
Fiber content: One medium pear contains 5.5 g of fiber.

- Pear

Pears are full of fiber, as well as vitamins C and A, folate and calcium. Keep a few pears in the fruit bowl, or serve them with dessert.

Fiber content: One medium pear contains 5.5 g of fiber.

- Apple

Apples are a good source of vitamins C and A and folate. Make sure to eat the skin as well as the apple flesh, as the skin contains much of the fruit's fiber.

Fiber content: One large apple contains 5.4 g of fiber.

- Raspberries

Raspberries are a great source of antioxidants. These ruby-red berries also contain vitamins C and K.

Fiber content: Half a cup of raspberries contains 4 g of fiber.

- Blackberries

Similarly to raspberries, blackberries are full of healthful antioxidants and are a great source of vitamins C and K.

Fiber content: Half a cup of blackberries contains 3.8 g of fiber.

- Prunes

Prunes, or dried plums, can help promote digestive health. Although high in fiber, prunes can also be high in sugar, so eat these in moderation.

Fiber content: Five prunes contain 3.4 g of fiber.

- Orange

Oranges are surprisingly a good source of fiber. Oranges are full of vitamin C, which is essential for health.

Fiber content: One orange contains 3.4 g of fiber.

- Banana

Bananas are a great source of nutrients, including potassium, magnesium, and vitamin C. They can be included in baking or eaten on their own as a snack.

Fiber content: One medium banana contains 3.1 g of fiber.

- Guava

Not only is this tropical fruit a source of fiber, but it also has a very high amount of vitamin C and contains vitamin A.

Try guava in smoothies or juices. The rinds are edible, which means they can make a great fruit snack when on the go.

Fiber content: One guava fruit contains 3 g of fiberTrusted Source

High-fiber nuts and seeds

Nuts and seeds provide numerous health benefits. They contain healthful fats, high concentrations of protein, and they often have essential omega-3 fatty acids.

High-fiber nuts and seeds include:

- Buckwheat

Buckwheat groats are grain-like seeds from a plant that is more closely related to rhubarb than wheat. It is rich in magnesium and zinc. Buckwheat does not contain gluten.

People traditionally use buckwheat in Japan for making soba noodles. It has also gained popularity in other countries.

People can add the groats to breakfast cereal or smoothies.

Buckwheat flour is an excellent gluten-free alternative to plain flour for baking and cooking.

Fiber content: Half a cup of buckwheat groats contains 8.4 g of fiber

- Chia seeds

People originally cultivated chia seeds in Central America. Not only are these edible seeds high in fiber, but they also contain high levels of omega-3s, protein, antioxidants, calcium, and iron.

People may get more health benefits from ground chia seeds. Buy them ground up or blitz the seeds into a fine powder, using a food processor or mortar and pestle.

Fiber content: Each tablespoon of chia seeds contains 4.1g of fiber.

- Quinoa

Quinoa is another pseudocereal and is also an edible seed.

This seed is high in antioxidants, magnesium, folate, and copper, as well as vitamins B-1, B-2, and B-6.

Quinoa is useful for people who are sensitive to gluten. Quinoa flour is excellent for baking, and people often include the flakes in breakfast cereals.

Fiber content: Half a cup of quinoa contains 2.6 g of fiber.

- Pumpkin seeds

Pumpkin seeds are a brilliant source of healthful monounsaturated and polyunsaturated fats, as well as magnesium, and zinc.

Fiber content: A quarter cup of pumpkin seeds contains 1.9 g of fibre.

- Almonds

Almonds are high in vitamin E, which acts as an antioxidant, as well as calcium and healthful, monounsaturated and polyunsaturated fatty acids.

Fiber content: Ten almonds contain 1.5 g of fiberTrusted Source

- Popcorn

Popcorn is a healthful, whole food snack. It is a source of zinc, folate, and vitamin A. Avoid popcorn brands high in sugar and salt.

Fiber content: One cup of popcorn contains 1.2 g of fiber

Whole grains

Whole grains help to keep the heart healthy and make people feel fuller after meals. High-fiber whole grains include:

- Freekeh

People make freekeh from roasted green wheat. They use it as a side to meat or mixed into salads to add substance and a nutty flavor.
Fiber content: Freekeh contains 13.3 g of fiber per 100 g.

- Bulgur wheat

Bulgur wheat is the whole-wheat grain popular in Middle Eastern cuisine. Processing bulgur wheat involves cracking the wheat germ open and parboiling it.

Bulgur wheat is a traditional ingredient in tabbouleh and pilafs. Use it as an alternative to rice in warm salads. Bear in mind that it is not gluten-free.
Fiber content: Bulgur wheat contains 4.5 g of fiber per 100 g.

- Pearled barley

Pearled barley is great as a side to meats, or in salads or stews.
Fiber content: Pearled barley contains 3.0g of fiber

High-fiber foods for a healthful diet
Medically reviewed by Katherine Marengo LDN, R.D. — Written by Cathleen Crichton-Stuart on September 21, 2018
Legumes
Vegetables
Fruit
Nuts and seeds
Whole grains
Tips to increase fiber in the diet
Summary
When a person includes high-fiber foods in their diet, it has many benefits, such as keeping the gut healthy, boosting heart health, and promoting weight loss.

According to the most up-to-date Dietary Guidelines for AmericansTrusted Source, the adequate intake (AI) of fiber for adult men is 33.6 grams (g) per day, and 28 g for adult women.

But most people in America do not meet this goal. The average fiber intake in the United States is 17 g, and only 5 percent of people meet the adequate daily intake.

People need to get both soluble and insoluble fiber from their diet. Eating a varied high-fiber diet means getting plenty of fruits, vegetables, legumes, and whole grains.

In this article, we provide a list of 38 healthful, high-fiber foods — explaining how much fiber each one has — to help people boost their daily fiber intake.

High-fiber nuts and seeds
Nuts and seeds provide numerous health benefits. They contain healthful fats, high concentrations of protein, and they often have essential omega-3 fatty acids.

High-fiber nuts and seeds include:

- Buckwheat

People can use buckwheat to make soba noodles.
Despite its name, buckwheat is a seed and not a grain.
Buckwheat groats are grain-like seeds from a plant that is more closely related to rhubarb than wheat. It is rich in magnesium and zinc. Buckwheat does not contain gluten.

People traditionally use buckwheat in Japan for making soba noodles. It has also gained popularity in other countries.
People can add the groats to breakfast cereal or smoothies.
Buckwheat flour is an excellent gluten-free alternative to plain flour for baking and cooking.
Fiber content: Half a cup of buckwheat groats contains 8.4 g of fiber

- Chia seeds

People originally cultivated chia seeds in Central America. Not only are these edible seeds high in fiber, but they also contain high levels of omega-3s, protein, antioxidants, calcium, and iron.

People may get more health benefits from ground chia seeds. Buy them ground up or blitz the seeds into a fine powder, using a food processor or mortar and pestle.
Fiber content: Each tablespoon of chia seeds contains 4.1g of fiber.

- Quinoa

Quinoa is another pseudocereal and is also an edible seed.

This seed is high in antioxidants, magnesium, folate, and copper, as well as vitamins B-1, B-2, and B-6.
Quinoa is useful for people who are sensitive to gluten. Quinoa flour is excellent for baking, and people often include the flakes in breakfast cereals.
Fiber content: Half a cup of quinoa contains 2.6 g of fiber.

- Pumpkin seeds

Pumpkin seeds are a brilliant source of healthful monounsaturated and polyunsaturated fats, as well as magnesium, and zinc.
Fiber content: A quarter cup of pumpkin seeds contains 1.9 g of fiber.

- Almonds

Almonds are high in vitamin E, which acts as an antioxidant, as well as calcium and healthful, monounsaturated and polyunsaturated fatty acids.
Fiber content: Ten almonds contain 1.5 g of fiber.

- Popcorn

Popcorn is a healthful, whole food snack. It is a source of zinc, folate, and vitamin A. Avoid popcorn brands high in sugar and salt.
Fiber content: One cup of popcorn contains 1.2 g of fiber.

Chapter twelve

Whole grains

Whole grains help to keep the heart healthy and make people feel fuller after meals. High-fiber whole grains include:

- Freekeh

People make freekeh from roasted green wheat. They use it as a side to meat or mixed into salads to add substance and a nutty flavor.
Fiber content: Freekeh contains 13.3 g of fiber per 100 g.

- Bulgur wheat

Bulgur wheat is the whole-wheat grain popular in Middle Eastern cuisine. Processing bulgur wheat involves cracking the wheat germ open and parboiling it.
Bulgur wheat is a traditional ingredient in tabbouleh and pilafs. Use it as an alternative to rice in warm salads. Bear in mind that it is not gluten-free.

Fiber content: Bulgur wheat contains 4.5 g of fiber per 100 g.

- Pearled barley

Pearled barley is great as a side to meats, or in salads or stews.
Fiber content: Pearled barley contains 3.8 g of fiber per 100 g.

Tips to increase fiber in the diet

The following tips can help people increase the amount of fiber they get in their diet each day:
Avoid peeling vegetables, as the skins contain plenty of fiber, including cellulose
swap white bread for wholemeal bread
swap white rice for brown rice
try using steel-cut or rolled oats instead of instant oats
aim for at least 2 ½ cupsTrusted Source of vegetables and 2 cupsTrusted Source of fruit each day.
choose starchy vegetables
use psyllium husk or other fiber supplements when unable to meet the adequate intake through diet

Fiber is an essential part of a healthful diet, though most people in the U.S. do not meet the recommended daily fiber intake.

A high-fiber diet helps to prevent constipation, maintain heart health, and feed the good bacteria in the gut. It can also help with weight loss.

BPeople can increase the amount of fiber they get from their diet by choosing high-fiber foods and following certain dietary tips, such as not peeling off edible skins on fruit and vegetables.

Foods that are naturally rich in fiber have many other health benefits, too. Eating a wide variety of whole foods will help people meet their daily needs for fiber and other key nutrients.

HEALTHFUL VEGETABLES

Eating plenty of vegetables can be one of the simplest ways to improve health and well-being. All vegetables contain healthful vitamins, minerals, and dietary fiber — but some stand out for their exceptional benefits.

Specific vegetables may offer more health advantages to certain people, depending on their diets, overall health, and nutritional needs.

Here are some vegetables listed below:

- Spinach is a leafy green vegetable and a great source of calcium, vitamins, iron, and antioxidants.

Due to its iron and calcium content, spinach is a great addition to any meat- or dairy-free diet.

One cup of raw spinach is mostly made up of water and contains only 7 caloriesTrusted Source. It also provides:

An adult's full daily requirementTrusted Source of vitamin K
high amounts of vitamin A
vitamin C
magnesium
folate
iron
calcium
antioxidants

Vitamin K is essential for a healthy body — especially for strong bones, as it improves the absorption of calcium.

Spinach also provides a good amount of iron for energy and healthy blood, and a high level of magnesium for muscle and nerve function.

It is also rich in antioxidants, and researchTrusted Source suggests that spinach leaves may lower blood pressure and benefit heart health.

If a person is taking blood thinners, such as warfarin (Coumadin), they should use caution when increasing their intake of dark leafy greens. Doctors recommend maintaining a consistent vitamin K intake over time for people taking these medications.

- How to eat spinach

People enjoy spinach raw in salads, sandwiches, and smoothies. Cooked spinach also has significant health benefits and is a great addition to pasta dishes and soups.

- Kale is a very popular leafy green vegetable with several health benefits. It provides around 7 caloriesTrusted Source per cup of raw leaves and good amounts of vitamins A, C, and K.

If a person is taking blood thinners, such as Coumadin, they should use caution when increasing their intake of dark leafy greens. It is best to maintain a consistent vitamin K intake while taking these medications.

How to eat kale

People use baby kale in pasta dishes, salads, and sandwiches. A person may also enjoy kale chips or juice.

- Broccoli is an incredibly healthful vegetable that belongs to the same family as cabbage, kale, and cauliflower. These are all cruciferous vegetables.

Each cup of chopped and boiled broccoli contains:
Around 31 caloriesTrusted Source
the full daily requirement of vitamin K
twice the daily recommended amount of vitamin C
According to the National Cancer InstituteTrusted Source, animal research has found that certain chemicals, called indoles and isothiocyanates, in cruciferous vegetables may inhibit the development of cancer in several organs, including the bladder, breasts, liver, and stomach.
These compounds may protect cells from DNA damage, inactivate cancer-causing agents, and have anti-inflammatory effects. However, research in humans has been mixed.

How to eat broccoli

Broccoli is very versatile. People can roast it, steam it, fry it, blend it into soups, or enjoy it warm in salads.
Peas are a sweet, starchy vegetable. They contain 134 caloriesTrusted Source per cooked cup, and they are rich in:
Fiber, providing 9(g) per serving
protein, providing 9g per serving
vitamins A, C, and K
Some certain B vitamins
Green peas are a good source of plant-based protein, which may be especially beneficial for people with vegetarian or vegan diets.

- Peas and other legumes contain fiber, which supports good bacteria in the gut and helps ensure regular bowel movements and a healthy digestive tract.

They are also rich in saponins, plant compounds that may help protect againstTrusted Source oxidative stress and cancer.

How to eat peas

It might be handy to keep a bag of peas in the freezer and gradually use them to boost the nutritional profiles of pasta dishes, risottos, and curries. A person might also enjoy a refreshing pea and mint soup.

- Sweet potatoes are root vegetables. Baked in its skin, a medium sweet potato provides 103 caloriesTrusted Source and 0.17 g of fat.

Each sweet potato also contains:much more than an adult's daily requirement of vitamin A
25% of their vitamin C and B6 requirements
12% of their potassium requirement

beta carotene, which may improve eye health and help fight cancer
Sweet potatoes may be a good option for people with diabetes. This is because they are low on the glycemic index and rich in fiber, so they may help regulate blood sugar.

How to eat sweet potatoes

For a simple meal, bake a sweet potato in its skin and serve it with a source of protein, such as fish or tofu.

- Beets

One cup of raw beets contains:
58.5 caloriesTrusted Source
442 milligrams (mg) of potassium
148 micrograms of folate
Beets and beet juice are great for improving heart health, as the vegetable is rich in heart-healthy nitrates. A small 2012 studyTrusted Source reports that drinking 500 g of beet juice significantly lowered blood pressure in healthy people.

These vegetables may also benefit people with diabetes. Beets contain an antioxidant called alpha-lipoic acid, which might be helpfulTrusted Source for people with diabetes-related nerve problems, called diabetic neuropathy.

How to eat beets

Roasting beets brings out their natural sweetness, but they also taste great raw in juices, salads, and sandwiches.

- Carrots

Each cup of chopped carrots contains 52 caloriesTrusted Source and over four times an adult's daily recommended intake of vitamin A, in the form of beta carotene.

Vitamin A is vital for healthy eyesight, and getting enough of this nutrient may help prevent vision loss.

Certain nutrients in carrots may also have cancer-fighting properties. A 2018 reviewTrusted Source of 10 articles reports that dietary carrot intake was associated with a reduced risk of breast cancer.

How to eat carrots

Carrots are extremely versatile. They work well in casseroles and soups, and they provide great health benefits when eaten raw, possibly with a dip such as hummus.

- Fermented vegetables

Fermented vegetables provide all the nutrients of their unfermented counterparts as well as healthful doses of probiotics.

Probiotics are beneficial bacteria that are present in the body and in some foods and supplements. Some researchers believe that they can improve gut health.

According to the National Center for Complementary and Integrative HealthTrusted Source, probiotics may help with symptoms of irritable bowel syndrome. They may also prevent infection- or antibiotic-induced diarrhea.

Some good vegetables for fermentation include:

.cabbage, as sauerkraut

.cucumbers, as pickles

.carrots

.cauliflower

How to eat fermented vegetables

People eat fermented vegetables in salads, sandwiches, or as a side dish.

- Tomatoes

Although tomatoes are technically a fruit, most people treat them like vegetables and use them in savory dishes. Each cup of chopped, raw tomatoes contains:

32 caloriesTrusted Source

427 mg of potassium

24.7 mg of vitamin C

Tomatoes contain lycopene, a powerful antioxidant. ResearchTrusted Source suggests that lycopene may help prevent prostate cancer, and the beta carotene in tomatoes also helps combat cancer.

Meanwhile, other potent antioxidants in tomatoes, such as lutein and zeaxanthin, may protect vision.

The Age-Related Eye Disease StudyTrusted Source reports that people who have high dietary intakes of these substances have a 25% reduced risk of age-related macular degeneration.

How to eat tomatoes

People enjoy tomatoes raw or cooked, and cooking them releases

All vegetables contain healthful vitamins, minerals, and dietary fiber but some stand out for their exceptional benefits.

Specific vegetables may offer more health advantages to certain people, depending on their diets, overall health, and nutritional needs.

In this article, we look at 15 of the most healthful vegetables and suggest ways to enjoy them as part of a balanced diet.

- Spinach

Andersen Ross/Getty Images.

Spinach is a leafy green vegetable and a great source of calcium, vitamins, iron, and antioxidants.

Due to its iron and calcium content, spinach is a great addition to any meat- or dairy-free diet.

One cup of raw spinach is mostly made up of water and contains only 7 caloriesTrusted Source. It also provides:

An adult's full daily requirementTrusted Source of vitamin K
high amounts of vitamin A
vitamin C
magnesium
folate
iron
calcium
antioxidants
Vitamin K is essential for a healthy body — especially for strong bones, as it improves the absorption of calcium.

Spinach also provides a good amount of iron for energy and healthy blood, and a high level of magnesium for muscle and nerve function.

It is also rich in antioxidants, and researchTrusted Source suggests that spinach leaves may lower blood pressure and benefit heart health.

If a person is taking blood thinners, such as warfarin (Coumadin), they should use caution when increasing their intake of dark leafy greens. Doctors recommend maintaining a consistent vitamin K intake over time for people taking these medications.

How to eat spinach

People enjoy spinach raw in salads, sandwiches, and smoothies. Cooked spinach also has significant health benefits and is a great addition to pasta dishes and soups.

- Kale

Kale is a very popular leafy green vegetable with several health benefits. It provides around 7 caloriesTrusted Source per cup of raw leaves and good amounts of vitamins A, C, and K.

Kale may benefit people with high cholesterol. One small 2008 study reports that males with high cholesterol who drank 150 milliliters of kale juice each day for 12 weeks experienced a 10% reduction in low-density lipoprotein, or "bad," cholesterol and a 27% increase in high-density lipoprotein, or "good," cholesterol.

If a person is taking blood thinners, such as Coumadin, they should use caution when increasing their intake of dark leafy greens. It is best to maintain a consistent vitamin K intake while taking these medications.

How to eat kale

People use baby kale in pasta dishes, salads, and sandwiches. A person may also enjoy kale chips or juice.

- Broccoli

Broccoli is an incredibly healthful vegetable that belongs to the same family as cabbage, kale, and cauliflower. These are all cruciferous vegetables.

Each cup of chopped and boiled broccoli contains:
Around 31 caloriesTrusted Source
the full daily requirement of vitamin K
twice the daily recommended amount of vitamin C
According to the National Cancer InstituteTrusted Source, animal research has found that certain chemicals, called indoles and isothiocyanates, in cruciferous vegetables may inhibit the development of cancer in several organs, including the bladder, breasts, liver, and stomach.

These compounds may protect cells from DNA damage, inactivate cancer-causing agents, and have anti-inflammatory effects. However, research in humans has been mixed.

How to eat broccoli

Broccoli is very versatile. People can roast it, steam it, fry it, blend it into soups, or enjoy it warm in salads.

For more science-backed resources on nutrition, visit our dedicated hub.

- Peas

Peas are a sweet, starchy vegetable. They contain 134 caloriesTrusted Source per cooked cup, and they are rich in:

fiber, providing 9 grams (g) per serving
protein, providing 9 g per serving
vitamins A, C, and K
certain B vitamins
Green peas are a good source of plant-based protein, which may be especially beneficial for people with vegetarian or vegan diets.

Peas and other legumes contain fiber, which supports good bacteria in the gut and helps ensure regular bowel movements and a healthy digestive tract.

They are also rich in saponins, plant compounds that may help protect againstTrusted Source oxidative stress and cancer.

How to eat peas

It might be handy to keep a bag of peas in the freezer and gradually use them to boost the nutritional profiles of pasta dishes, risottos, and curries. A person might also enjoy a refreshing pea and mint soup.

- Sweet potatoes

Guido Mieth/Getty Images.
Sweet potatoes are root vegetables. Baked in its skin, a medium sweet potato provides 103 caloriesTrusted Source and 0.17 g of fat.

Each sweet potato also contains:

much more than an adult's daily requirement of vitamin A
25% of their vitamin C and B6 requirements
12% of their potassium requirement
beta carotene, which may improve eye health and help fight cancer
Sweet potatoes may be a good option for people with diabetes. This is because they are low on the glycemic index and rich in fiber, so they may help regulate blood sugar.

How to eat sweet potatoes

For a simple meal, bake a sweet potato in its skin and serve it with a source of protein, such as fish or tofu.

- Beets

One cup of raw beets contains:

58.5 caloriesTrusted Source
442 milligrams (mg) of potassium
148 micrograms of folate
Beets and beet juice are great for improving heart health, as the vegetable is rich in heart-healthy nitrates. A small 2012 studyTrusted Source reports that drinking 500 g of beet juice significantly lowered blood pressure in healthy people.

These vegetables may also benefit people with diabetes. Beets contain an antioxidant called alpha-lipoic acid, which might be helpfulTrusted Source for people with diabetes-related nerve problems, called diabetic neuropathy.

How to eat beets

Roasting beets brings out their natural sweetness, but they also taste great raw in juices, salads, and sandwiches.

- Carrots

Each cup of chopped carrots contains 52 caloriesTrusted Source and over four times an adult's daily recommended intake of vitamin A, in the form of beta carotene.

Vitamin A is vital for healthy eyesight, and getting enough of this nutrient may help prevent vision loss.

Certain nutrients in carrots may also have cancer-fighting properties. A 2018 reviewTrusted Source of 10 articles reports that dietary carrot intake was associated with a reduced risk of breast cancer.

How to eat carrots
Carrots are extremely versatile. They work well in casseroles and soups, and they provide great health benefits when eaten raw, possibly with a dip such as hummus.

- Fermented vegetables

Fermented vegetables provide all the nutrients of their unfermented counterparts as well as healthful doses of probiotics.

Probiotics are beneficial bacteria that are present in the body and in some foods and supplements. Some researchers believe that they can improve gut health.

According to the National Center for Complementary and Integrative HealthTrusted Source, probiotics may help with symptoms of irritable bowel syndrome. They may also prevent infection- or antibiotic-induced diarrhea.

Some good vegetables for fermentation include:

cabbage, as sauerkraut
cucumbers, as pickles
carrots
cauliflower
How to eat fermented vegetables
People eat fermented vegetables in salads, sandwiches, or as a side dish.

9. Tomatoes
Although tomatoes are technically a fruit, most people treat them like vegetables and use them in savory dishes. Each cup of chopped, raw tomatoes contains:

32 caloriesTrusted Source
427 mg of potassium
24.7 mg of vitamin C
Tomatoes contain lycopene, a powerful antioxidant. ResearchTrusted Source suggests that lycopene may help prevent prostate cancer, and the beta carotene in tomatoes also helps combat cancer.

Meanwhile, other potent antioxidants in tomatoes, such as lutein and zeaxanthin, may protect vision.

The Age-Related Eye Disease StudyTrusted Source reports that people who have high dietary intakes of these substances have a 25% reduced risk of age-related macular degeneration.

How to eat tomatoes

People enjoy tomatoes raw or cooked, and cooking them releases more lycopene.

- Garlic

People have long used garlic in cooking and medicine. Each garlic clove contains just 4 caloriesTrusted Source and is low in vitamins and minerals.

However, garlic is a natural antibiotic. For example, a 2018 reviewTrusted Source notes that people have used garlic for purposes similar to those of antibiotics since the 16th century.

Allium, a component of garlic, may be the source of its health benefits. Confirming this will require more research.

How to eat garlic

Heating garlic reduces its health benefits, so it is best to eat garlic raw, in bruschetta or dips, for example.

What are the most healthful vegetables?

Eating plenty of vegetables may be one of the simplest ways to improve health and well-being.

All vegetables contain healthful vitamins, minerals, and dietary fiber — but some stand out for their exceptional benefits.

Specific vegetables may offer more health advantages to certain people, depending on their diets, overall health, and nutritional needs.

In this article, we look at 15 of the most healthful vegetables and suggest ways to enjoy them as part of a balanced diet.

- Spinach

Andersen Ross/Getty Images.

Spinach is a leafy green vegetable and a great source of calcium, vitamins, iron, and antioxidants.

Due to its iron and calcium content, spinach is a great addition to any meat- or dairy-free diet.

One cup of raw spinach is mostly made up of water and contains only 7 caloriesTrusted Source. It also provides:

An adult's full daily requirementTrusted Source of vitamin K
high amounts of vitamin A
vitamin C
magnesium
folate

iron
calcium
antioxidants
Vitamin K is essential for a healthy body — especially for strong bones, as it improves the absorption of calcium.

Spinach also provides a good amount of iron for energy and healthy blood, and a high level of magnesium for muscle and nerve function.

It is also rich in antioxidants, and researchTrusted Source suggests that spinach leaves may lower blood pressure and benefit heart health.

If a person is taking blood thinners, such as warfarin (Coumadin), they should use caution when increasing their intake of dark leafy greens. Doctors recommend maintaining a consistent vitamin K intake over time for people taking these medications.

How to eat spinach
People enjoy spinach raw in salads, sandwiches, and smoothies. Cooked spinach also has significant health benefits and is a great addition to pasta dishes and soups.

- Kale

Kale is a very popular leafy green vegetable with several health benefits. It provides around 7 caloriesTrusted Source per cup of raw leaves and good amounts of vitamins A, C, and K.

Kale may benefit people with high cholesterol. One small 2008 study reports that males with high cholesterol who drank 150 milliliters of kale juice each day for 12 weeks experienced a 10% reduction in low-density lipoprotein, or "bad," cholesterol and a 27% increase in high-density lipoprotein, or "good," cholesterol.

Research from 2015Trusted Source, meanwhile, suggests that kale juice can reduce blood pressure, blood cholesterol, and blood sugar levels.

If a person is taking blood thinners, such as Coumadin, they should use caution when increasing their intake of dark leafy greens. It is best to maintain a consistent vitamin K intake while taking these medications.

How to eat kale
People use baby kale in pasta dishes, salads, and sandwiches. A person may also enjoy kale chips or juice.

- Broccoli

Broccoli is an incredibly healthful vegetable that belongs to the same family as cabbage, kale, and cauliflower. These are all cruciferous vegetables.

Each cup of chopped and boiled broccoli contains:
Around 31 caloriesTrusted Source
the full daily requirement of vitamin K
twice the daily recommended amount of vitamin C
According to the National Cancer InstituteTrusted Source, animal research has found that certain chemicals, called indoles and isothiocyanates, in cruciferous vegetables may inhibit the development of cancer in several organs, including the bladder, breasts, liver, and stomach.

These compounds may protect cells from DNA damage, inactivate cancer-causing agents, and have anti-inflammatory effects. However, research in humans has been mixed.

How to eat broccoli
Broccoli is very versatile. People can roast it, steam it, fry it, blend it into soups, or enjoy it warm in salads.

For more science-backed resources on nutrition, visit our dedicated hub.

- Peas

Peas are a sweet, starchy vegetable. They contain 134 caloriesTrusted Source per cooked cup, and they are rich in:

fiber, providing 9 grams (g) per serving
protein, providing 9 g per serving
vitamins A, C, and K
certain B vitamins
Green peas are a good source of plant-based protein, which may be especially beneficial for people with vegetarian or vegan diets.
Peas and other legumes contain fiber, which supports good bacteria in the gut and helps ensure regular bowel movements and a healthy digestive tract.

They are also rich in saponins, plant compounds that may help protect againstTrusted Source oxidative stress and cancer.

How to eat peas
It might be handy to keep a bag of peas in the freezer and gradually use them to boost the nutritional profiles of pasta dishes, risottos, and curries. A person might also enjoy a refreshing pea and mint soup.

- Sweet potatoes

Guido Mieth/Getty Images.
Sweet potatoes are root vegetables. Baked in its skin, a medium sweet potato provides 103 caloriesTrusted Source and 0.17 g of fat.

Each sweet potato also contains:

much more than an adult's daily requirement of vitamin A
25% of their vitamin C and B6 requirements
12% of their potassium requirement
beta carotene, which may improve eye health and help fight cancer
Sweet potatoes may be a good option for people with diabetes. This is because they are low on the glycemic index and rich in fiber, so they may help regulate blood sugar.

How to eat sweet potatoes
For a simple meal, bake a sweet potato in its skin and serve it with a source of protein, such as fish or tofu.

- Beets

One cup of raw beets contains:

58.5 caloriesTrusted Source
442 milligrams (mg) of potassium
148 micrograms of folate
Beets and beet juice are great for improving heart health, as the vegetable is rich in heart-healthy nitrates. Drinking 500 g of beet juice significantly lowered blood pressure in healthy people.

These vegetables may also benefit people with diabetes. Beets contain an antioxidant called alpha-lipoic acid, which might be helpfulTrusted Source for people with diabetes-related nerve problems, called diabetic neuropathy.

How to eat beets

Roasting beets brings out their natural sweetness, but they also taste great raw in juices, salads, and sandwiches.

- Carrots

Each cup of chopped carrots contains 52 caloriesTrusted Source and over four times an adult's daily recommended intake of vitamin A, in the form of beta carotene.
Vitamin A is vital for healthy eyesight, and getting enough of this nutrient may help prevent vision loss.

Certain nutrients in carrots may also have cancer-fighting properties. Dietary carrot intake was associated with a reduced risk of breast cancer.

How to eat carrots
Carrots are extremely versatile. They work well in casseroles and soups, and they provide great health benefits when eaten raw, possibly with a dip such as hummus.

- Fermented vegetables

Fermented vegetables provide all the nutrients of their unfermented counterparts as well as healthful doses of probiotics.

Probiotics are beneficial bacteria that are present in the body and in some foods and supplements. Some researchers believe that they can improve gut health.

According to the National Center for Complementary and Integrative HealthTrusted Source, probiotics may help with symptoms of irritable bowel syndrome. They may also prevent infection- or antibiotic-induced diarrhea.

Some good vegetables for fermentation include:

cabbage, as sauerkraut
cucumbers, as pickles
carrots
cauliflower
How to eat fermented vegetables

People eat fermented vegetables in salads, sandwiches, or as a side dish.

- Tomatoes

Although tomatoes are technically a fruit, most people treat them like vegetables and use them in savory dishes. Each cup of chopped, raw tomatoes contains:

32 caloriesTrusted Source
427 mg of potassium
24.7 mg of vitamin C
Tomatoes contain lycopene, a powerful antioxidant. ResearchTrusted Source suggests that lycopene may help prevent prostate cancer, and the beta carotene in tomatoes also helps combat cancer.

Meanwhile, other potent antioxidants in tomatoes, such as lutein and zeaxanthin, may protect vision.

The Age-Related Eye Disease StudyTrusted Source reports that people who have high dietary intakes of these substances have a 25% reduced risk of age-related macular degeneration.

How to eat tomatoes

People enjoy tomatoes raw or cooked, and cooking them releases more lycopene.

- Garlic

People have long used garlic in cooking and medicine. Each garlic clove contains just 4 caloriesTrusted Source and is low in vitamins and minerals.

However, garlic is a natural antibiotic. For example, a 2018 reviewTrusted Source notes that people have used garlic for purposes similar to those of antibiotics since the 16th century.

Allium, a component of garlic, may be the source of its health benefits. Confirming this will require more research.

How to eat garlic

Heating garlic reduces its health benefits, so it is best to eat garlic raw, in bruschetta or dips, for example.

- Onions

Each cup of chopped onions can provideTrusted Source:
64 calories
vitamin C
vitamin B6
manganese
Onions and other allium vegetables, including garlic, contain sulfur compounds. Review studies, including a 2019 reviewTrusted Source and a 2015 reviewTrusted Source, suggest that these compounds may help protect against cancer.

How to eat onions

It can be easy to incorporate onions into soups, stews, stir-fries, and curries. To get the most from their antioxidants, eat them raw — in sandwiches, salads, and dips such as guacamole.

- Alfalfa sprouts

Each cup of alfalfa sprouts contains only 8 caloriesTrusted Source and a good amount of vitamin K.

These sprouts also boast several compounds that contribute to good health, including:
Saponins, a type of bitter compound with health benefits
flavonoids, a type of polyphenol known for its anti-inflammatory and antioxidant effects
phytoestrogens, plant compounds that are similar to natural estrogens
Traditionally, some have used alfalfa sprouts to treat a range of health conditions, such as arthritis and kidney problems. However, very few scientific investigations have explored these uses.

Research suggests that alfalfa sprouts contain antioxidants, which are compounds that may help fight diseases including cancer and heart disease.

Eating sprouted legumes such as these may have other benefits. StudiesTrusted Source suggest that sprouting, or germinating, seeds increases their protein and amino acid contents.

Germination may also improveTrusted Source the digestibility of alfalfa and other seeds and increase their dietary fiber content.

How to eat alfalfa sprouts

People enjoy alfalfa sprouts in salads and sandwiches.

- Bell peppers

Sweet bell peppers may be red, yellow, or orange. Unripe, green bell peppers are also popular, though they taste less sweet.

A cup of chopped red bell pepper provides:

39 caloriesTrusted Source

190 mg of vitamin C

0.434 mg of vitamin B6

folate

beta carotene, which the body converts into vitamin A

Antioxidants and bioactive chemicals present in bell peppers includeTrusted Source:

Ascorbic acid

carotenoids

vitamin C

beta carotene

flavonoids, such as quercetin and kaempferol

How to eat bell peppers

Bell peppers are extremely versatile and can be easy to incorporate into pasta, scrambled eggs, or a salad. A person might also enjoy them sliced with a side of guacamole or hummus.

- Cauliflower

One cup of chopped cauliflower contains:

27 caloriesTrusted Source

plenty of vitamin C

vitamin K

fiber

Eeating 25 g of dietary fiber each day to promote heart and gut health.

Also, cauliflower and other cruciferous vegetables contain an antioxidant called indole-3-carbinol. ResearchTrusted Source has linked this compound with cancer-combatting effects in animals. However, confirming the effects in humans requires more research.

And like broccoli, cauliflower contains another compound that may help combat cancer: sulforaphane.

How to eat cauliflower

A person can pulse raw cauliflower in a blender to make cauliflower rice or turn it into a pizza base for a low-calorie, comforting treat. People may also enjoy cauliflower in curries or baked with olive oil and garlic.

- Seaweed

Seaweed, also known as sea vegetables, are versatile and nutritious plants that provide several health benefits. Common Types of seaweed include:
kelp
nori
sea lettuce
spirulina
wakame
Seaweed is one of the few plant-based sources of the omega-3 fatty acids docosahexaenoic acid and eicosapentaenoic acid. These are essential for health and are mostly present in meat and dairy.

Each type of seaweed has a slightly different nutritional profile, but they are typically rich in iodine, which is an essential nutrient for thyroid function.

Eating a variety of sea vegetables can provide the body with several important antioxidants to reduce cellular damage.

Also, many types of seaweed contain chlorophyll, which is a plant pigment that has anti-inflammatory propertiesTrusted Source.

Brown sea vegetables, such as kelp and wakame, contain another potent antioxidant called fucoxanthin. ResearchTrusted Source suggests that this has 13.5 times the antioxidant power of vitamin E.

How to eat seaweed

When possible, choose organic seaweed and eat small amounts to avoid introducing too much iodine into the diet. People enjoy sea vegetables in sushi, miso soups, and as a seasoning for other dishes.

Eating vegetables every day is important for health. They provide essential vitamins, minerals, and other nutrients, such as antioxidants and fiber.

People who eat at least 5 servings of vegetables a day have the lowest risk of many diseases, including cancer and heart disease.

Enjoy a range of vegetables daily to reap as many health benefits as possible.

DISCUSSION QUESTIONS

Do you like to eat fruits? What's your favorite one?
How often do you eat fresh fruit?
In your opinion, what's the most delicious fruit?
Do you like vegetables? What's your favorite one?
Do you think that fruits and vegetables are good for your health? Why or why not?
Are you or would you like to be vegetarian?
How often do you drink fruit juice? What kind of fruit juice do you drink?
Do you like to eat fruit salad?
What kind of vegetables and fruits do you buy at the supermarket?
What the means the saying: "An apple a day keeps the doctor away?"
What are the most common fruits and vegetables in your country?
Can fruits and vegetables help you cure diseases?
Can fruits and vegetables help you lose weight if you are on a diet?
Do you cultivate fruits or vegetables in your garden?
Do you like to use things that have a fruit smell? (E.g: Perfumes, erasers, etc)
What's the most delicious fruit in your opinion?
Do you think that fruits and vegetables are good for your health? Why (not)?
Are you / would you like to be vegetarian?
How many vegetables and fruits do you buy at the supermarket?
What is the meaning of the saying: "An apple a day keeps the doctor away?"
What are the most common fruits and vegetables in your country?

www.ingramcontent.com/pod-product-compliance
Lightning Source LLC
LaVergne TN
LVHW080558160826
845677LV00010B/1900

* 9 7 9 8 8 4 8 0 3 7 8 1 4 *